YOUR KNOWLEDGE HAS VALUE

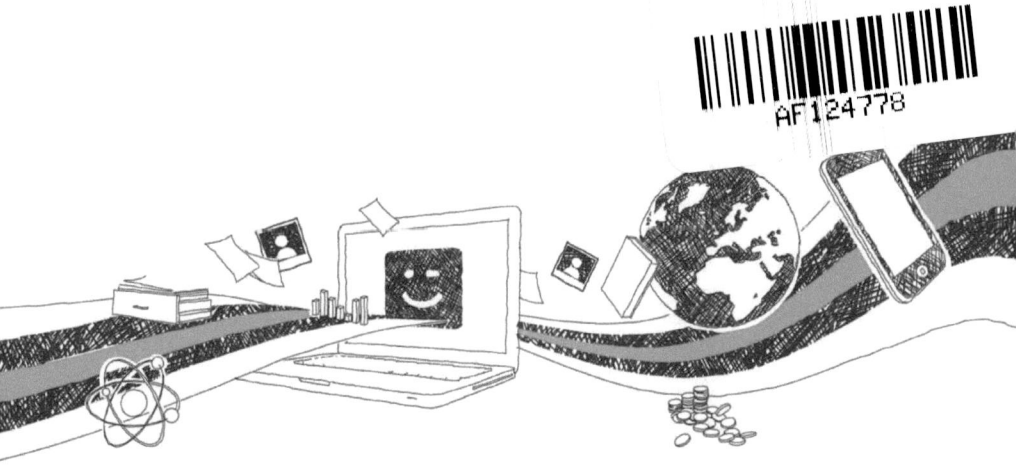
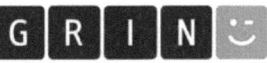

Bibliographic information published by the German National Library:

The German National Library lists this publication in the National Bibliography; detailed bibliographic data are available on the Internet at http://dnb.dnb.de .

Imprint:

Copyright © 2016 GRIN Verlag, Open Publishing GmbH
Print and binding: Books on Demand GmbH, Norderstedt Germany
ISBN: 9783668335219

This book at GRIN:

http://www.grin.com/en/e-book/341493/in-silico-analysis-and-modeling-of-delete-rious-single-nucleotide-polymorphism

Marwa Osman, et al.

In Silico Analysis and Modeling of Deleterious Single Nucleotide Polymorphism (Snps) in Human GATA4 Gene

GRIN Publishing

GRIN - Your knowledge has value

Since its foundation in 1998, GRIN has specialized in publishing academic texts by students, college teachers and other academics as e-book and printed book. The website www.grin.com is an ideal platform for presenting term papers, final papers, scientific essays, dissertations and specialist books.

Visit us on the internet:

http://www.grin.com/

http://www.facebook.com/grincom

http://www.twitter.com/grin_com

In Silico Analysis and Modeling of Deleterious Single Nucleotide Polymorphism (Snps) in Human *GATA4* Gene

Mojahed A. Alhag [1*], Marwa M. Osman[1*], Soada A. Osman [2], Sara A. Elsanosi [1], Salma M. Elwakeel [3], Asma A. Mohamed [1], Mosab M. Gasemelseed [1], Aisha I. Ibrahim[1] , Zhoor A. Ahmed [4] & Mohamed A. Salih[1]

[1] Department of Biotechnology, Africa city of Technology- Khartoum, Sudan
[2] Sudan Medical Council - Khartoum, Sudan
[3] Taha Basheer Psychatric Hospital- Khartoum, Sudan
[4] Al-Neelain University-Faculty of Pharmacy- Khartoum, Sudan

Corresponding author: Marwa Mohamed Osman
*Contributed equally

ABSTRACT

Congenital heart disease (CHD) presents as the abnormality in the structure and function of heart and great vessels caused by embryonic development disorders, it is highly complex and is not fully understood yet. This study aimed to perform a computational analysis of the nsSNPs in the *GATA4* gene, to identify the possible mutations and propose a modeled structure for the mutant protein that potentially affects its function. The nsSNPs were analyzed using 5 prediction tools: SIFT, Polyphen-2, I-Mutant 3.0, PhD-SNP and Project Hope. While the SNPs on 3'UTR and 5'UTR regions were analyzed using PolymRTS and SNP Function Prediction softwares, respectively. Twenty nine nsSNPs were found to be deleterious and damaging by SIFT and 22 nsSNPs by PolyPhen server; 22 nsSNPs were found to be common in both SIFT and PolyPhen server. Also, 6 nsSNPs were observed to be highly deleterious and damaging as per SIFT and PolyPhen server. Moreover the PolymiRTS results showed 34 SNPs in the 3'UTR region and only one SNP in 5' UTR by SNP Function Prediction to be functionally significant. Hence, we hope our results will provide useful information that needed to help researchers to do further study in heart disease in children especially in our country.

Keywords: Congenital heart disease (CHD), SNP, *GATA4* and SNP Function Prediction.

Table of Contents

INTRODUCTION

Congenital heart disease (CHD) affects approximately 1.33 million of the newborns in United States and worldwide, Defects of atrial and ventricular septation are the most frequent form of congenital heart disease, accounting for almost 50% of all cases. CHD presents as the abnormality in the structure and function of heart and great vessels caused by embryonic development disorders, it is highly complex and is not fully understood yet [1-6].

A single nucleotide polymorphism (SNP) is a single base mutation in DNA, as an alternative form of sequence variation for gene identification and mapping studies also can consider genetic markers, SNPs can be used to follow the inheritance patterns of chromosomal regions from generation to generation and are powerful tools in the study of genetic factors associated with human diseases among these non-synonymous single nucleotide polymorphisms (nsSNPs) that lead to an amino acid change in the protein product are of particular interest for their close relevance to human inherited diseases Functional impacts of nsSNPs generally fall into two classes: disease-associated (deleterious) and benign (no observable phenotypic effect). [7-9]

The human a zinc finger protein*GATA4* gene maps to chromosome 8p23.1-p22, consists of seven exons, and encodes a protein of 442 amino acids (MIM n600576), is consider one of the hypertrophy-responsive transcription factors is expressed in adult vertebrate heart, gut epithelium, and gonads. During fetal development *GATA4* is expressed in yolk sac endoderm and cells involved in heart formation. *GATA-4* forms a functional protein complex with an intrinsic histone acetyltransferase, p300 and regulates pathological cardiac hypertrophy. Disruption of this complex result in the inhibition of cardiac hypertrophy and heart failure in vivo .*GATA-4* play an important role in embrognatic heart development also may regulate a set of cardiac-specific genes and play a crucial role in cardiogenesis such as develop of right ventricle, numerous cardiac gene, including myosin heavy chin (±- MHC), cardiac troponin-C(C-TNC) and a trial natriuretic factor have been shown to be direct transcription target *GATA4* a rounding more than 1,700 gene have been reported to be involved in the development. also is the most important gene change causes the phenotype atrial Septal defect, (ASD) which accounts for about 33% of all congenital cardiovascular deformities, affecting over 3 out of 1,000 live births. [10-21]

Furthermore severe forms of congenital heart disease, including septation defects, outflow tract alignment defects, dextrocardia, pulmonary stenosis and chamber hypoplasia observed in patients with *GATA4* mutation or deletion in which indicate GATA4 is an important regulator of cardiomyocyte proliferation through direct transcriptional activation of cell cycle regulators, including cyclin D2 and cdk4.[22-24]

3

In addition reduction in dosage of *GATA4* leads to abnormal cardiac development with a common atrioventricular canal, double outlet right ventricle, and hypoplasia of the ventricular myocardium.[13]

In the present study we aimed to perform a computational analysis of the nsSNPs in the *GATA4* gene, to identify the possible mutations and propose a modeled structure for the mutant protein that potentially affects its function.

Materials and Methods

Dataset

Human *GATA4* gene data were obtained from OMIM (#600576 - http://www.ncbi.nlm.nih.gov/omim) and Entered on the National Center for Biotechnology Information (NCBI) website in December 2015, including Protein accession number (NP_002043) and mRNA accession number (NM_002052). The Uniprot accession number (P43694) was obtained in the Swissprot database (http://expasy.org). The information of SNPs in human *GATA4* was collected from dbSNP (http://www.ncbi.nlm.nih.gov/snp). Gene's functions and other genes that related to *GATA4* gene were obtained from GeneMANIA (http://www.genemania.org/).

Functional analysis Prediction

The nsSNPs were analyzed using 5 prediction tools: SIFT, Polyphen-2, I-Mutant 3.0, PANTHER, SNPs3D, PhD-SNP and Project Hope while the SNPs on 3'UTR and 5'UTR regions were analyzed using PolymRTS and SNP Function Prediction softwares, respectively, Figure (1). The data for amino acid sequence of the human *MC1R* gene (ref. Seq. NP_002043), Uniprot accession number (P43694), position in the protein, and wild and mutated residue of the nsSNPs were used according to the program requirements.

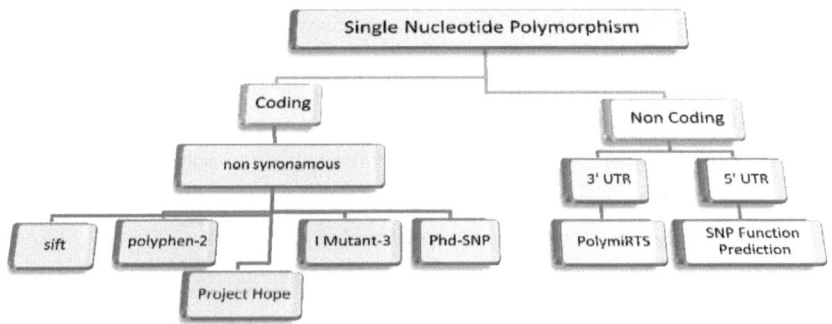

Figure (1): Softwares used in our investigation

SIFT software (http://sift.bii.a-star.edu.sg/). This is a sequences homology-based tool that presumes that important amino acids will be conserved in the protein family. Hence, changes at well-conserved positions tend to be predicted as deleterious [25]. The cutoff value in the SIFT program is a tolerance index of ≥0.05. The higher the tolerance index, the less functional impact a particular amino acid substitution is likely to have.

PolyPhen-2 (Polymorphism Phenotyping v2). This server is available at http://genetics.bwh.harvard.edu/pph2/ has been used to analyze the structural damage due to coding nsSNPs which can affect protein functionality. The server is able to calculate a score on the basis of the characterization of the substitution site to a known protein three-dimensional structure. A PSIC score has been calculate for each variant of each site and the difference between them reported. The higher the PSIC score difference is, the higher is the functional impact a particular amino acid substitution is likely to have. PolyPhen scores were assigned probably damaging (2.00 or more), possibly damaging (1.40–1.90), potentially damaging (1.0–1.50), benign (0.00–0.90). Basically PolyPhen accepts input in form of SNPs or protein sequences [26].

I Mutant 3.0 is a support vector machine (SVM) tool for the prediction of protein stability free-energy change (ΔΔG or DDG) on a specific nsSNP. It predicts the free energy changes starting from either the protein structure or the protein sequence. A negative DDG value means that the mutation decreases the stability of the protein, while a positive DDG value indicates an

5

increase in stability. I-Mutant 3.0 also implements a prediction of disease-associated SNPs from a sequence analysis based on a decision tree with the SVM-based classifier (SVM-Sequence) coupled to the SVM-Profile trained on sequence profile information. The nsSNPs are then classified as disease-related or neutral polymorphisms [27].

PhD-SNP (Predictor of Human Deleterious Single Nucleotide Polymorphisms) is a SVM-based classifier that uses protein sequence information to predict whether an nsSNP is disease-associated, based on a supervised training algorithm. The output is obtained from the frequencies of the wild and mutant residues, the number of aligned sequences, and the conservation index alculated for the position involved, and provides a prediction of disease-related (disease) or neutral polymorphism [28].

Project Hope software (http://www.cmbi.ru.nl/hope/input) is an online web service where the user can submit a sequence and mutation. This software collects structural information from a series of sources, including calculations on the 3D protein structure, sequence annotations in UniProt and predictions from DAS-servers. It combines this information to give analyze the effect of a certain mutation on the protein structure and will show the effect of that mutation in such a way that even those without a bioinformatics background can understand it [29].

PolymiRTS is a database of naturally occurring DNA variations in microRNA seed regions and microRNA target sites. Integrated data from CLASH (cross linking, ligation and sequencing of hybrids) experiments, PolymiRTS database provides more complete and accurate microRNA–mRNA interactions [31]. The polymorphic microRNA target sites are assigned into four classes: 'D' (the derived allele disrupts a conserved microRNA site), 'N' (the derived allele disrupts a nonconserved microRNA site), 'C' (the derived allele creates a new microRNA site) and 'O' (other cases when the ancestral allele cannot be determined unambiguously). The class 'C' may cause abnormal gene repression and class 'D' may cause loss of normal repression control. So these two classes of PolymiRTS are most likely to have functional impacts [30-31]. PolymiRTS is available at (http://compbio.uthsc.edu/miRSNP/).

SNP Function Prediction (https://snpinfo.niehs.nih.gov/cgibin/snpinfo/snpfunc.cgi) SNP function prediction (FuncPred) checked if the SNP variants could alter transcriptional regulation by affecting transcription factor binding sites (TFBS) activity or changing of splicing pattern or efficiency by disrupting splice site, exonic splicing enhancers (ESE) or silencers (ESS).

GeneMANIA (http://www.genemania.org/) is an online database that helps you predict the function of your favorite genes and gene sets. GeneMANIA finds other genes that are related to a set of input genes, using a very large set of functional association data. Association data include protein and genetic interactions, pathways, co-expression, co-localization and protein domain similarity. You can use GeneMANIA to find new members of a pathway or complex, find additional genes you may have missed in your screen or find new genes with a specific function, such as protein kinases. Your question is defined by the set of genes you input [32].

RESULTS

According to NCBI database (http://www.ncbi.nlm.nih.gov/projects/SNP); The *GATA4* gene contained a total of 18598 SNPs at the time of the study, out of which 5982 were *Homo sapiens,* 120 occurred in coding synonymous SNPs, 192 occurred in nsSNPs, 147 occurred in the miRNA 3' UTR, 334 occurred in 5' UTR region, 5 occurred in Frame Shift and 5486 occurred in intronic regions. We selected (missense & nonsense) nsSNPs, 3' UTR and 5' UTR SNPs for our investigation.

Prediction Programs

A total of 192 nsSNPs from the NCBI dbSNP database were analyzed to identify the deleterious mutations by SIFT software. Of these, 26 (59 mutatios) were found to be damaging (score < 0.05), with 12 assigned a score of 0.

In Polyphen-2, a total of 22 nsSNPs (in 51 mutations) were predicted as damaging (PSIC > 0.5); 6 of these nsSNPs were predicted to be highly deleterious, with a PSIC score of 1.

The DDG predicted by I-Mutant 3.0 classified 18 (41 mutations) of the nsSNPs as decreasing the stability of the mutated protein (DDG <0) and 5(10 mutatios) as increasing it (DDG=00.4 to -0.25).

The PhD-SNP 2.0 tool classified the mutation as a disease-related or neutral polymorphism. Of the set of nsSNPs in the *GATA4* gene analyzed, 11 (22 mutations) were predicted to be disease-related by PhD-SNP 2.0 and the 11 SNPs (22 mutations) predicted to be Neutral. The prediction results of the 5 tools are summarized in Table (1).

Highest deleterious nature among these damaging nsSNPs of *GATA4* gene obtained from previously described software and addition to I mutant /Phd-SNP server presented to Project Hope (http://www.cmbi.ru.nl/hope/input) revealed the 3D structure for the truncated proteins with its new candidates; in addition, it described the reaction and physiochemical properties of these candidates. Here we present the results upon each candidate and discus the conformational variations and interactions with the neighboring amino acids, Figure (2) illuminates these six highest SNPs. The sequences of The Transcription factor (GATA-4) protein (and its 2 isofroms) were obtained from ExPASy Database (www.expasy.org/).

In PolymiRTS software, a total of 167 SNPs at 3'UTR were analyzed and only 34 were predicted by this software, Table (2).

In SNP Function Prediction; the output showed that among 334 SNPs at 5'UTR region of *GATA-4* gene, only one SNPs was predicted, namely rs61277615, Table (3).

The Transcription factor (GATA-4) protein had many vital functions. Gene's functions and the genes co-expressed with, share similar protein domain, or participate to achieve similar function are illustrated by using GeneMANIA and shown in Table (4), Table (5).

Table (1): list of nonsynonymous SNPs with SIFT, POLYPHEN-2, I MUTAT AD PHD-SNP results.

SNP	CHR/ Coordinate	Nucleotide Change	Amino Acid Change	Sift Prediction	Sift Score	Polyphen-2 Result	PSIC SD	RI	DDG value	SVM2	R	Prediction
rs1139240	8/11565876	G/C	E19Q	Deleterious (Warning Low Confidence)	0	Probably Damaging	0.997	1	-0.28	Decrease	4	Neutral
rs1139241	8/11565936	G/C	V39L	Deleterious	0.008	Probably Damaging	0.958	5	-0.87	Decrease	3	Neutral
rs56208331	8/11615928	G/A	D425N	Deleterious	0.008	Probably Damaging	0.97	3	-0.89	Decrease	8	Neutral
rs56208331	8/11615928	G/A	D426N	Deleterious	0.008	Probably Damaging	0.97	3	-0.89	Decrease	8	Neutral
rs56298569	8/11612591	C/G	Q316E	Deleterious	0	Probably Damaging	0.996	1	-0.43	Decrease	2	Disease
rs56298569	8/11612591	C/G	Q110E	Deleterious	0	Probably Damaging	0.995	1	-0.43	Decrease	2	Disease
rs56298569	8/11612591	C/G	Q317E	Deleterious	0	Possibly Damaging	0.784	1	-0.43	Decrease	2	Disease
rs104894074	8/11565975	C/T	S52F	Deleterious	0.002	Probably Damaging	0.975	0	-0.25	Increase	3	Disease
rs116430078	8/11607693	C/T	A286V	Deleterious	0.037	Possibly Damaging	0.892	1	-0.07	Decrease	0	Neutral
rs116430078	8/11607693	C/T	A287V	Deleterious	0.037	Possibly Damaging	0.676	1	-0.07	Decrease	0	Neutral
rs138404762	8/11612576	C/T	R311W	Deleterious	0	Probably Damaging	0.999	5	-0.34	Decrease	7	Disease
rs138404762	8/11612576	C/T	R105W	Deleterious	0	Probably Damaging	0.997	5	-0.34	Decrease	7	Disease

rs138404762	8/11612576	C/T	R312W	Deleterious	0	Probably Damaging	0.997	5	-0.34	Decrease	7	Disease
rs145999237	8/11614530	C/T	R362C	Deleterious	0.029	Probably Damaging	1	3	-0.71	Increase	1	Neutral
rs145999237	8/11614530	C/T	R363C	Deleterious	0.03	Probably Damaging	1	3	-0.71	Increase	1	Neutral
rs145999237	8/11614530	C/T	R156C	Deleterious	0.04	Probably Damaging	1	3	-0.71	Increase	2	Neutral
rs146017816	8/11615980	C/G	A442G	Deleterious (Warning Low Confidence)	0	Probably Damaging	0.999	7	-1.12	Decrease	8	Neutral
rs146017816	8/11615980	C/G	A236G	Deleterious (Warning Low Confidence)	0	Probably Damaging	0.997	7	-1.12	Decrease	8	Neutral
rs146017816	8/11615980	C/G	A443G	Deleterious (Warning Low Confidence)	0	Probably Damaging	0.997	7	-1.12	Decrease	8	Neutral
rs146017816	8/11615980	C/T	A442V	Deleterious (Warning Low Confidence)	0	Probably Damaging	0.999	0	0.12	Increase	8	Neutral
rs146017816	8/11615980	C/T	A236V	Deleterious (Warning Low Confidence)	0	Probably Damaging	0.999	0	0.12	Increase	8	Neutral
rs146017816	8/11615980	C/T	A443V	Deleterious	0	Probably Damaging	0.999	0	0.12	Increase	8	Neutral

rs ID	Position	Alleles	Variant	SIFT	SIFT score	PolyPhen	PolyPhen score		Stability	Effect		Classification
rs149351193	8/11615967	G/T	D438Y	Deleterious (Warning Low Confidence)	0.009	Probably Damaging	0.969	0	0.08	Increase	0	Disease
rs149351193	8/11615967	G/T	D439Y	Deleterious (Warning Low Confidence)	0.009	Probably Damaging	0.969	0	0.08	Increase	0	Disease
rs180765750	8/11607684	G/A	R283H	Deleterious	0	Probably Damaging	1	5	-0.81	Decrease	7	Disease
rs180765750	8/11607684	G/A	R77H	Deleterious	0	Probably Damaging	1	5	-0.81	Decrease	7	Disease
rs180765750	8/11607684	G/A	R284H	Deleterious	0	Probably Damaging	1	6	-0.92	Decrease	7	Disease
rs199922907	8/11565833	C/T	A6V	Deleterious (Warning Low Confidence)	0	Probably Damaging	0.986	1	0.04	Decrease	5	Neutral
rs202213149	8/11565883	G/T	G21V	Deleterious	0.017	Probably Damaging	0.963	4	0.04	Increase	3	Neutral
rs267601735	8/11606487	C/G	P226A	Deleterious	0	Probably Damaging	1	9	-1.6	Decrease	8	Disease
rs267601735	8/11606487	C/G	P20A	Deleterious	0	Probably Damaging	0.999	9	-1.6	Decrease	8	Disease
rs267601735	8/11606487	C/G	P227A	Deleterious	0	Probably Damaging	1	9	-1.6	Decrease	8	Disease
rs368091578	8/11606580	C/T	P257S	Deleterious	0	Probably Damaging	0.987	8	-1.53	Decrease	8	Disease
rs368091578	8/11606580	C/T	P258S	Deleterious	0	Possibly Damaging	0.753	8	-1.53	Decrease	8	Disease

rs368091578	8/11606580	C/T	P51S	Deleterious	0.007	Probably Damaging	0.991	8	-1.53	Decrease	8	Disease
rs370946998	8/11606448	G/C	E7Q	Deleterious	0.005	Probably Damaging	0.998	8	-0.74	Decrease	7	Disease
rs370946998	8/11606448	G/C	E213Q	Deleterious	0.009	Possibly Damaging	0.875	8	-0.88	Decrease	8	Disease
rs374132087	8/11565829	A/C	Q3P	Deleterious (Warning Low Confidence)	0	Probably Damaging	0.996	5	-0.29	Decrease	2	Neutral
rs377222076	8/11612585	G/A	G108R	Deleterious	0.001	Probably Damaging	0.998	3	-0.35	Decrease	5	Disease
rs377222076	8/11612585	G/A	G314R	Deleterious	0.003	Probably Damaging	0.999	3	-0.35	Decrease	4	Disease
rs377222076	8/11612585	G/A	G315R	Deleterious	0.003	Probably Damaging	0.969	3	-0.35	Decrease	4	Disease
rs377673676	8/11606439	G/A	D210N	Deleterious	0.01	Probably Damaging	0.996	4	-1.22	Decrease	3	Neutral
rs377673676	8/11606439	G/A	D211N	Deleterious	0.011	Probably Damaging	1	4	-1.21	Decrease	3	Neutral
rs377673676	8/11606439	G/A	D4N	Deleterious	0.032	Probably Damaging	1	2	-0.94	Decrease	4	Neutral
rs387906770	11565948	C/T	R43W	Deleterious	0	Probably Damaging	1	3	-0.53	Decrease	1	Neutral
rs387906771	11607675	C/T	T280M	Deleterious	0	Probably Damaging	1	4	0.02	Decrease	4	Disease
rs387906771	11607675	C/T	T74M	Deleterious	0	Probably Damaging	1	4	0.02	Decrease	5	Disease
rs387906771	11607675	C/T	T281M	Deleterious	0	Probably Damaging	1	4	0.02	Decrease	4	Disease
rs387906772	11612573	A/G	M310V	Deleterious	0	Possibly Damaging	0.934	7	-0.6	Decrease	7	Disease

| rs387906772 | 11612573 | A/G | M311V | Deleterious | 0 | Possibly Damaging | 0.618 | 7 | -0.6 | Decrease | 6 | Disease |
| rs387906772 | 11612573 | A/G | M104V | Deleterious | 0.002 | Possibly Damaging | 0.946 | 7 | -0.6 | Decrease | 6 | Disease |

PolyPhen-2 result: POROBABLY DAMAGING (more confident prediction) / POSSIBLY DAMAGING (less confident prediction), **PSIC SD:** Position-Specific Independent Counts software if the score is ≥ 0.5, **Tolerance Index:** Ranges from 0 to 1. The amino acid substitution is predicted damaging if the score is ≤ 0.05, and tolerated if the score is > 0.05. **RI**: Reliability Index **DDG**: $\Delta\Delta G$ sign **SVM**: support vector machine **DDG value:** DG (New Protein)-DG (Wild Type) in Kcal/mole, **SVM2 value:** DDG < 0: decrease stability, DDG >0 increase stability.

13

SNP ID	3D Structure	Amino Acid Change
rs56298569		Mutation of glutamine into a glutamic acid at position 316
rs138404762		Mutations of an arginine into a tryptophan at positions 105, 311 and 312
rs180765750		Mutations of an arginine into a histidine at positions 77, 283 and 284
rs267601735		Mutations of a proline into a alanine at positions 20, 226 and 227
rs377222076		Mutations of a glycine into a arginine at position 108
rs387906771		Mutations of a threonine into a arginine at positions 74, 280 and 281

Figure (2): 3D model by Project Hope for GATA4 proteins

Location	dbSNP ID	Wobble base pair	Ancestral Allele	Allele	miR ID	Conservation	miRSite	Function Class	context+ score change
11615993	rs185843389	N	C	C	hsa-miR-6077	2	ttccCTCTTCCct	D	No Change
					hsa-miR-6873-5p	2	tTCCCTCTtcct	D	No Change
				T	hsa-miR-4668-5p	9	ttccCTTTTCCCt	C	No Change
					hsa-miR-5584-5p	10	ttccctTTTCCCT	C	No Change
					hsa-miR-6124	2	ttccCTTTTCCct	C	No Change
11616015	rs148278615	N	C	C	hsa-miR-1973	3	ccTGCACGGAcct	D	-0.482
				T	hsa-miR-5581-3p	3	cctGCATGGAcct	C	-0.184
					hsa-miR-6872-3p	3	cctGCATGGAcct	C	-0.132
11616122	rs3729857	N	G	C	hsa-miR-4444	8	cttgAACTCGAca	C	-0.229
11616164	rs7459940	N	G	G	hsa-miR-3200-5p	1	ttCTCAGATgcct	N	-0.144
					hsa-miR-4251	1	TTCTCAGAtgcct	N	-0.288
					hsa-miR-4329	1	tTCTCAGAtgcct	N	-0.096
					hsa-miR-6761-5p	1	tTCTCAGAtgcct	N	-0.09

11616338				C	hsa-miR-3607-5p	2	ttcTCACATGcct	C	-0.13
	rs867858	N	A	A	hsa-miR-2117	2	GAGAACAagcgga	D	-0.034
					hsa-miR-4273	2	GAGAACAAgcgga	D	-0.144
					hsa-miR-4677-5p	2	gAGAACAAgcgga	D	0.008
					hsa-miR-6739-3p	2	gAGAACAAgcgga	D	0.035
					hsa-miR-7156-5p	2	GAGAACAAgcgga	D	-0.144
				C	hsa-miR-152-5p	2	gAGAACCAgcgga	C	-0.044
					hsa-miR-182-3p	2	gAGAACCAgcgga	C	-0.05
					hsa-miR-597-3p	2	GAGAACCAgcgga	C	-0.247
11616349	rs78334561	N	C	C	hsa-miR-1538	1	gagggCCGGGCCc	N	-0.215
					hsa-miR-4745-3p	1	gagggCCGGGCCc	N	-0.205
				T	hsa-miR-4687-5p	1	GAGGGCTgggccc	C	-0.097
11616382	rs188654804	N	C	A	hsa-miR-1298-5p	1	GAATGAAggcatc	C	-0.112
					hsa-miR-205-5p	1	gaATGAAGGcatc	C	-0.07

16

Position	rsID	N	Allele	miRNA		Sequence	Code	Value
				hsa-miR-4297	1	gaatGAAGGCAtc	C	-0.098
				hsa-miR-532-5p	2	gaatgAAGGCATc	C	-0.065
				hsa-miR-5581-5p	1	gaatGAAGGCAtc	C	-0.101
11616398	rs7008652	N	T	hsa-miR-4802-3p	2	ttgCCATGTAcct	D	-0.059
				hsa-miR-942-3p	1	ttGCCATGTAcct	N	-0.349
			C	hsa-miR-3688-5p	2	TTGCCACgtacct	C	-0.112
11616465	rs181138914	N	C	hsa-miR-3141	2	tggcaCCGCCCTg	D	-0.226
				hsa-miR-4746-3p	2	tgGCACCGCcctg	D	-0.22
			T	hsa-miR-34a-5p	2	tggCACTGCCctg	C	-0.101
				hsa-miR-34c-5p	2	tggCACTGCCctg	C	-0.101
				hsa-miR-4436b-3p	2	tggcaCTGCCCTg	C	-0.125
				hsa-miR-449a	2	tggCACTGCCctg	C	-0.092
				hsa-miR-449b-5p	2	tggCACTGCCctg	C	-0.092
				hsa-miR-4632-5p	2	tggcaCTGCCCTg	C	-0.134
				hsa-miR-6735-5p	2	tggcaCTGCCCTg	C	-0.134
				hsa-miR-6879-5p	2	tggcaCTGCCCTg	C	-0.134
				hsa-miR-7843-5p	2	tggcaCTGCCCTg	C	-0.144
11616501	rs884662	N	C	hsa-miR-4328	5	ccAAAACTGtggg	D	0.029
11616516	rs904018	N	T	hsa-miR-297	1	gtgACATACAAgt	N	-0.085
				hsa-miR-3149	1	gtgaCATACAAgt	N	No Change
				hsa-miR-567	1	gtgACATACAAgt	N	-0.033
				hsa-miR-643	1	gtgacATACAAGt	N	-0.013

					hsa-miR-675-3p	1	gtgaCATACAAgt	N	-0.033
				C	hsa-miR-147a	1	gtgaCACACAAgt	C	-0.023
					hsa-miR-581	1	gtgacACACAAGt	C	-0.041
					hsa-miR-592	1	gTGACACAcaagt	C	-0.067
					hsa-miR-597-5p	1	GTGACACAcaagt	C	-0.26
					hsa-miR-6818-5p	1	gtgaCACACAAgt	C	-0.039
					hsa-miR-6867-5p	1	gtgACACACAagt	C	-0.042
11616529	rs1062221	Y	A	A	hsa-miR-124-5p	1	gacTGAACACttc	N	-0.055
					hsa-miR-4255	2	gactGAACACTtc	D	-0.081
				G	hsa-miR-302a-3p	2	gactgAGCACTTc	C	-0.005
					hsa-miR-302b-3p	2	gactgAGCACTTc	C	-0.005
					hsa-miR-302c-3p	2	gactgAGCACTTc	C	-0.005
					hsa-miR-302d-3p	2	gactgAGCACTTc	C	-0.005
					hsa-miR-302e	2	gactgAGCACTTc	C	-0.015
					hsa-miR-372-3p	2	gactgAGCACTTc	C	-0.005
					hsa-miR-373-3p	2	gactgAGCACTTc	C	-0.015
					hsa-miR-3934-3p	1	gaCTGAGCActtc	C	-0.067
					hsa-miR-4264	1	GACTGAGcacttc	C	-0.123
					hsa-miR-520a-3p	2	gactgAGCACTTc	C	-0.024
					hsa-miR-520b	2	gactgAGCACTTc	C	-0.005
					hsa-miR-520c-3p	2	gactgAGCACTTc	C	-0.005
					hsa-miR-520d-3p	2	gactgAGCACTTc	C	-0.024
					hsa-miR-520e	2	gactgAGCACTTc	C	-0.015

11616547	rs12825	N	G	C	hsa-miR-210-5p	0	gagctaCAGGGGC	C	-0.226
					hsa-miR-3137	0	gaGCTACAGgggc	C	-0.075
					hsa-miR-1251-5p	0	gaGCTAGAGgggc	N	-0.091
					hsa-miR-4749-3p	0	gagctaGAGGGGC	N	-0.273
11616570	rs185327204	N	C	C	hsa-miR-5008-3p	3	ccacAGCACAGcc	D	-0.07
					hsa-miR-6737-3p	3	ccacAGCACAGcc	D	-0.042
					hsa-miR-7157-3p	3	ccacAGCACAGcc	D	-0.051
					hsa-miR-7974	21	ccacagCACAGCC	D	-0.1
					hsa-miR-4318	1	CCACAGTAcagcc	C	-0.213
					hsa-miR-4693-5p	1	cCACAGTAcagcc	C	-0.014
					hsa-miR-4718	3	ccacaGTACAGCc	C	-0.118
					hsa-miR-892a	1	cCACAGTAcagcc	C	-0.038
11616571	rs804291	Y	G	A	hsa-miR-5008-3p	3	cacAGCACAGcct	C	-0.07
					hsa-miR-6737-3p	3	cacAGCACAGcct	C	-0.042
					hsa-miR-7157-3p	3	cacAGCACAGcct	C	-0.051
					hsa-miR-7974	21	cacagCACAGCCt	C	-0.1

19

Position	rsID	Y/N	Allele 1	Allele 2	miRNA	#	Sequence	Class	Value
11616792	rs191109800	Y	G	A	hsa-miR-191-3p	3	cacAGCGCAGcct	D	-0.155
					hsa-miR-604	21	cacagcCGCAGCCt	D	-0.157
			A		hsa-miR-1257	0	cccttCATTCACc	N	-0.041
					hsa-miR-3179	0	CCCTTCAttcacc	N	-0.043
					hsa-miR-6864-5p	0	CCCTTCAttcacc	N	-0.114
					hsa-miR-7515	0	CCCTTCAttcacc	N	-0.056
11616835	rs141296821	N	T	C	hsa-miR-589-3p	2	acaaaaTGTTCTG	C	-0.076
11616836	rs804290	Y	A	G	hsa-miR-19a-5p	2	CAAAACAttctgc	C	0.031
					hsa-miR-19b-1-5p	2	CAAAACAttctgc	C	0.031
					hsa-miR-19b-2-5p	2	CAAAACAttctgc	C	0.031
					hsa-miR-2052	2	CAAAACAttctgc	C	0.035
					hsa-miR-33a-3p	2	caAAACATTctgc	C	0.069
					hsa-miR-4307	2	cAAAACATtctgc	C	0.081
11616870	rs146304341	Y	G	G	hsa-miR-1587	2	cactCAGCCCAgc	D	-0.1
					hsa-miR-3620-5p	2	cactCAGCCCAgc	D	-0.1
					hsa-miR-378g	2	cactcAGCCCAGc	D	-0.077
					hsa-miR-4492	2	cactCAGCCCAgc	D	-0.064
					hsa-miR-4498	2	cactCAGCCCAgc	D	-0.061

					hsa-miR-4656	2	cacTCAGCCCAgc	D	-0.189
					hsa-miR-4675	2	cactCAGCCCAgc	D	-0.084
					hsa-miR-4741	2	cactCAGCCCAgc	D	-0.07
					hsa-miR-5001-5p	2	cactCAGCCCAgc	D	-0.061
					hsa-miR-6829-5p	2	cactCAGCCCAgc	D	-0.066
					hsa-miR-762	2	cactCAGCCCAgc	D	-0.061
					hsa-miR-8077	2	cACTCAGCccagc	D	-0.014
				A	hsa-miR-1238-5p	2	CACTCAAccagc	C	-0.039
					hsa-miR-3940-5p	2	cactCAACCCAgc	C	-0.07
					hsa-miR-4507	2	cactCAACCCAgc	C	-0.07
					hsa-miR-4658	2	CACTCAAccagc	C	-0.039
					hsa-miR-4758-5p	2	CACTCAAccagc	C	-0.029
					hsa-miR-5589-5p	2	cactcaACCCAGC	C	-0.128
					hsa-miR-6790-5p	2	CACTCAAccagc	C	-0.035
11616963	rs182365313	G	N	G	hsa-miR-1324	2	CTGTCTGtctgct	D	-0.049
					hsa-miR-3166	1	ctgtcTGTCTGCt	N	-0.061
				C	hsa-miR-4524a-3p	2	CTGTCTCtctgct	C	-0.016
11616996	rs139566390	C	N	C	hsa-miR-149-5p	1	tggcAGCCAGAgt	N	-0.061
					hsa-miR-3064-5p	1	tggCAGCCAGAgt	N	-0.183

21

				miR		Sequence		Value
				hsa-miR-4794	1	tggcAGCCAGAgt	N	-0.057
				hsa-miR-514a-5p	1	tggcagCCAGAGT	N	-0.051
				hsa-miR-604	1	tgGCAGCCAgagt	N	-0.138
				hsa-miR-647	1	tgGCAGCCAgagt	N	-0.114
				hsa-miR-6504-5p	1	tggCAGCCAGAgt	N	-0.183
				hsa-miR-664a-5p	1	tggcAGCCAGAgt	N	-0.057
				hsa-miR-6762-3p	1	tgGCAGCCAgagt	N	-0.122
		T		hsa-miR-301a-5p	1	tggcaGTCAGAGt	C	-0.067
				hsa-miR-345-5p	1	tggcAGTCAGAgt	C	-0.03
				hsa-miR-4714-5p	1	tggcagTCAGAGT	C	0.003
				hsa-miR-5002-3p	1	tGGCAGTCAgagt	C	-0.409
		C		hsa-miR-4649-5p	1	cagCTCGCCCcg	N	-0.155
				hsa-miR-485-5p	2	CAGCCTCgccccg	D	-0.037
				hsa-miR-6729-5p	1	cagcCTCGCCCcg	N	-0.174
				hsa-miR-6884-5p	2	CAGCCTCgccccg	D	-0.055
		T		hsa-miR-4708-3p	2	caGCCTTGCccg	C	-0.109
				hsa-miR-5090	0	cagcctTGCCCCG	C	-0.222
				hsa-miR-6775-5p	0	cagcctTGCCCCG	C	-0.232
				hsa-miR-6809-5p	2	cagCCTTGCCccg	C	-0.069

11617022   rs187432043   N   C

22

					miRNA		Sequence		
11617023	rs144191832	Y	G	G	hsa-miR-4649-5p	1	agcCTCGCCCcgg	N	-0.155
					hsa-miR-6729-5p	1	agcCTCGCCCcgg	N	-0.174
					hsa-miR-6784-5p	0	agcctcGCCCGG	N	-0.236
			A		hsa-miR-2467-5p	2	AGCCTCAccccgg	C	-0.065
					hsa-miR-3188	2	AGCCTCAccccgg	C	-0.064
					hsa-miR-3975	2	AGCCTCAccccgg	C	-0.069
					hsa-miR-4316	2	aGCCTCACcccgg	C	-0.127
					hsa-miR-4710	2	agCCTCACCCcgg	C	-0.107
					hsa-miR-485-5p	2	AGCCTCAccccgg	C	-0.143
					hsa-miR-6884-5p	2	AGCCTCAccccgg	C	-0.146
11617082	rs146102045	N	C	G	hsa-miR-2115-5p	1	cgaatTGGAAGCA	C	-0.349
					hsa-miR-516a-3p	1	cgaatcGGAAGCA	C	-0.133
					hsa-miR-516b-3p	1	cgaattGGAAGCA	C	-0.133
					hsa-miR-7162-5p	1	cgaatcGGAAGCA	C	-0.133
11617120	rs114395528	N	G	G	hsa-miR-3124-3p	2	tGGAAAGAagacg	D	-0.023
					hsa-miR-4778-3p	1	tggaAAGAAGAcg	N	0.029

11617142	rs11785481	N	C	C	hsa-miR-6740-3p	1	tggaaAGAAGACg	N	-0.117
					hsa-miR-6752-3p	2	acacGGCAGGGgg	D	-0.123
					hsa-miR-6801-3p	1	acacgGCAGGGGg	N	-0.12
					hsa-miR-6810-3p	1	acacgGCAGGGGg	N	-0.13
				T	hsa-miR-3162-3p	2	acacGGTAGGGgg	C	-0.128
11617145	rs115161018	N	G	G	hsa-miR-6752-3p	2	cGGCAGGGggggcc	D	-0.123
					hsa-miR-6801-3p	1	cgGCAGGGGgggcc	N	-0.12
					hsa-miR-6810-3p	1	cgGCAGGGGgggcc	N	-0.13
11617181	rs191938369	N	C	C	hsa-miR-1203	1	ctGCTCCGGgatc	N	-0.253
					hsa-miR-6081	2	CTGCTCCgggatc	D	-0.09
				T	hsa-miR-2278	2	CTGCTCTgggatc	C	-0.055
					hsa-miR-6501-3p	1	cTGCTCTGggatc	C	-0.044
11617192	rs139741267	Y	G	G	hsa-miR-6820-5p	1	tCTGCCGCgttct	N	-0.269
11617240	rs12458	N	T	T	hsa-miR-136-5p	0	agctcATGGAGAc	N	-0.065
					hsa-miR-556-5p	0	AGCTCATggagac	N	-0.068

24

Position	rs#		Allele	Allele	miRNA	No.	Sequence		Score
11617252	rs76841597	N	C	C	hsa-miR-3125	4	ctccTTCCTCTtt	D	-0.071
					hsa-miR-3916	4	ctccTTCCTCTtt	D	-0.062
					hsa-miR-4476	1	ctCCTTCCTctt	N	-0.13
					hsa-miR-4533	1	cTCCTTCCtctt	N	-0.113
					hsa-miR-583	1	ctccttCTCTTT	N	-0.1
					hsa-miR-6859-5p	4	ctccTTCCTCTtt	D	-0.081
					hsa-miR-6876-5p	1	ctCCTTCCTctt	N	-0.121
			T		hsa-miR-4311	4	ctcctttCTCTTT	C	-0.08
11617339	rs10622770	Y	G	G	hsa-miR-187-5p	9	ctggcTGTAGCAg	D	-0.122
					hsa-miR-221-3p	9	ctggcTGTAGCAg	D	-0.111
					hsa-miR-222-3p	9	ctggcTGTAGCAg	D	-0.114
					hsa-miR-548v	8	ctggCTGTAGCAg	D	-0.334
					hsa-miR-6856-3p	8	ctGGCTGTAgcag	D	-0.148
					hsa-miR-3651	8	ctGGCTATAgcag	C	-0.142
11617365	rs3735812	Y	A	A	hsa-miR-4676-5p	7	CTGGCTAtagcag	C	-0.194
					hsa-miR-575	7	CTGGCTAtagcag	C	-0.195
					hsa-miR-6858-3p	7	CTGGCTAtagcag	C	-0.146
					hsa-miR-6813-3p	9	aCCAAGGTtctgt	C	-0.258
11617422	rs149831548	N	C	C	hsa-miR-1321	2	taCCTCCCTAac	D	-0.383
					hsa-miR-149-3p	3	taCCCTCCtaac	D	-0.316

25

hsa-miR-3162-5p	2	taccCTCCCTAAc	D	-0.36
hsa-miR-4728-5p	3	taCCCTCCCtaac	D	-0.298
hsa-miR-4739	2	taccCTCCCTAAac	D	-0.425
hsa-miR-4756-5p	2	taccCTCCCTAAc	D	-0.393
hsa-miR-6760-5p	2	taccCTCCCTAAc	D	-0.143
hsa-miR-6785-5p	3	taCCCTCCCtaac	D	-0.288
hsa-miR-6883-5p	3	taCCCTCCCtaac	D	-0.279
hsa-miR-1207-5p	3	taCCCTGCCtaac		
hsa-miR-1910-3p	2	taccCTGCCTAAc		
hsa-miR-2682-5p	2	taccCTGCCTAAc		
hsa-miR-34b-5p	2	taccCTGCCTAAc		
hsa-miR-4423-3p	6	taccCTGCCTAAc		
hsa-miR-449c-5p	2	taccCTGCCTAAc		
hsa-miR-4763-3p	3	taCCCTGCCtaac		
hsa-miR-6511a-5p	2	taccCTGCCTAAc		

G

hsa-miR-6808-5p	2	tacCCTGCCTAac
hsa-miR-6893-5p	2	tacCCTGCCTAac
hsa-miR-940	2	tacCCTGCCTAac

Table (2): SNPs and INDELs in miRNA target sites at 3'UTR by PolymiRTS Software

'D': the derived allele disrupts a conserved microRNA site, **'N'**: the derived allele disrupts a nonconserved microRNA site, **'C'**: the derived allele creates a new microRNA site.

Table (3): SNP in Transcriptional factor binding sites and splicing site on *GATA4* gene at 5'UTR by SNP Function Prediction

dbSNP ID	Chromosome	Position	Allele	TFBS	Splicing(site)	(ESE or ESS)
rs61277615	8	11599137	C/T	Y	--	--

TFBS: Transcription factor-binding site **ESE:** exonic splicing enhancer **ESS:** exonic splicing silencer

Table (4): the *GATA4* functions and its appearance in network and genome

Feature	FDR	Genes in network	Genes in genome
cardiac chamber morphogenesis	1.01E-11	8	60
stem cell differentiation	1.01E-11	10	171
heart morphogenesis	1.80E-11	9	120
cardiac chamber development	1.86E-11	8	70
cardiac septum development	2.28E-11	7	37
ventricular septum development	1.30E-10	6	21
cardiac ventricle development	3.62E-10	7	56
cardiac septum morphogenesis	5.30E-10	6	27
heart development	6.76E-10	9	202
cardiocyte differentiation	6.76E-10	7	64
muscle structure development	3.19E-09	9	244
cardiac atrium morphogenesis	4.07E-09	5	15
cardiac muscle tissue development	4.07E-09	7	85
cardiac ventricle morphogenesis	1.08E-08	6	47
cardiac atrium development	1.35E-08	5	19
striated muscle tissue development	1.21E-07	7	142
epithelial to mesenchymal transition	1.21E-07	6	71
embryonic organ development	1.26E-07	7	144
muscle tissue development	1.59E-07	7	150
negative regulation of cell differentiation	1.96E-07	8	266
regulation of pathway-restricted SMAD protein phosphorylation	2.65E-07	5	35
pathway-restricted SMAD protein phosphorylation	4.48E-07	5	39
atrial septum development	6.15E-07	4	13

blood vessel development	7.40E-07	7	193
ventricular septum morphogenesis	7.92E-07	4	14
tissue morphogenesis	1.32E-06	7	212
transmembrane receptor protein serine/threonine kinase signaling pathway	1.54E-06	7	218
chordate embryonic development	2.17E-06	6	125
embryo development ending in birth or egg hatching	2.17E-06	6	125
smooth muscle cell differentiation	2.46E-06	4	19
cardioblast differentiation	2.46E-06	4	19
regulation of transmembrane receptor protein serine/threonine kinase signaling pathway	2.73E-06	6	132
muscle cell differentiation	5.95E-06	6	151
BMP signaling pathway	1.10E-05	5	79
mesenchyme development	1.14E-05	5	80
pattern specification process	1.78E-05	6	184
outflow tract morphogenesis	2.16E-05	4	33
columnar/cuboidal epithelial cell differentiation	3.02E-05	4	36
vasculogenesis	3.68E-05	4	38
negative regulation of cell motility	5.79E-05	5	116
positive regulation of stem cell differentiation	5.79E-05	3	10
negative regulation of cell migration	5.79E-05	5	114
regulation of transcription initiation from RNA polymerase II promoter	5.79E-05	3	10
receptor serine/threonine kinase binding	5.79E-05	3	10
cardiac right ventricle morphogenesis	5.79E-05	3	10
negative regulation of cellular component movement	6.71E-05	5	120
regulation of DNA-templated transcription, initiation	7.46E-05	3	11
cardiac muscle cell differentiation	7.83E-05	4	48
sequence-specific DNA binding	8.82E-05	6	254
regulation of nervous system development	8.85E-05	6	255
negative regulation of locomotion	9.03E-05	5	130
epithelial cell differentiation	1.02E-04	6	263
regulatory region DNA binding	1.05E-04	6	267
transcription regulatory region DNA binding	1.05E-04	6	266
regulatory region nucleic acid binding	1.05E-04	6	267
regulation of cardiac muscle cell proliferation	1.08E-04	3	13

regulation of vasculature development	1.44E-04	5	146
mesenchymal cell development	1.61E-04	4	60
regulation of cardiac muscle tissue growth	1.64E-04	3	15
negative regulation of binding	1.66E-04	4	61
negative regulation of cellular component organization	1.85E-04	6	299
mesenchymal cell differentiation	2.50E-04	4	68
blood vessel morphogenesis	2.64E-04	5	170
regulation of stem cell differentiation	2.64E-04	4	70
cardiac muscle cell proliferation	2.64E-04	3	18
striated muscle cell proliferation	2.64E-04	3	18
muscle organ development	2.76E-04	5	172
regulation of heart growth	3.01E-04	3	19
heart valve development	3.44E-04	3	20
heart valve morphogenesis	3.44E-04	3	20
cardiac muscle tissue growth	3.95E-04	3	21
embryonic morphogenesis	4.30E-04	5	191
regulation of muscle cell differentiation	4.30E-04	4	81
skeletal system development	4.75E-04	5	196
cardiac muscle cell development	4.98E-04	3	23
sequence-specific DNA binding RNA polymerase II transcription factor activity	4.99E-04	5	199
cardiac cell development	5.91E-04	3	25
regulation of cardiac muscle tissue development	5.91E-04	3	25
stem cell development	5.91E-04	4	90
negative regulation of BMP signaling pathway	5.91E-04	3	25
regulation of organ growth	5.91E-04	3	25
positive regulation of pathway-restricted SMAD protein phosphory-lation	5.91E-04	3	25
heart growth	6.59E-04	3	26
regionalization	8.02E-04	4	98
regulation of neurogenesis	8.50E-04	5	227
striated muscle cell differentiation	8.63E-04	4	101
negative regulation of multicellular organismal process	8.63E-04	5	229
embryonic organ morphogenesis	8.63E-04	4	101
dorsal/ventral pattern formation	1.27E-03	3	33
organ growth	1.27E-03	3	33

heart looping	1.38E-03	3	34
determination of heart left/right asymmetry	1.49E-03	3	35
cardiac muscle tissue morphogenesis	1.87E-03	3	38
embryonic heart tube morphogenesis	1.87E-03	3	38
regulation of binding	1.99E-03	4	127
muscle organ morphogenesis	2.12E-03	3	40
muscle tissue morphogenesis	2.12E-03	3	40
embryonic heart tube development	2.59E-03	3	43
regulation of BMP signaling pathway	2.59E-03	3	43
in utero embryonic development	3.36E-03	3	47
digestive tract development	3.55E-03	3	48
determination of left/right symmetry	3.69E-03	3	49
regulation of protein complex assembly	3.69E-03	4	152
digestive system development	3.69E-03	3	49
morphogenesis of an epithelium	4.36E-03	4	159
positive regulation of transmembrane receptor protein ser-ine/threonine kinase signaling pathway	4.56E-03	3	53
muscle cell proliferation	4.74E-03	3	54
determination of bilateral symmetry	4.74E-03	3	54
specification of symmetry	4.92E-03	3	55
regulation of developmental growth	4.92E-03	3	55
regulation of striated muscle tissue development	5.15E-03	3	56
tube development	5.19E-03	4	169
regulation of muscle tissue development	5.28E-03	3	57
regulation of osteoblast differentiation	5.28E-03	3	57
regulation of muscle organ development	5.52E-03	3	58
striated muscle cell development	6.06E-03	3	60
transcription initiation from RNA polymerase II promoter	7.70E-03	4	189
regulation of vasculogenesis	8.18E-03	2	10
co-SMAD binding	8.18E-03	2	10
muscle cell development	8.53E-03	3	68
negative regulation of cell development	9.23E-03	3	70
outflow tract septum morphogenesis	9.74E-03	2	11
DNA-templated transcription, initiation	1.13E-02	4	212
heart trabecula morphogenesis	1.13E-02	2	12
cardiac left ventricle morphogenesis	1.13E-02	2	12

cardiac epithelial to mesenchymal transition	1.13E-02	2	12
negative regulation of transmembrane receptor protein ser-ine/threonine kinase signaling pathway	1.22E-02	3	78
osteoblast differentiation	1.35E-02	3	81
aorta morphogenesis	1.52E-02	2	14
regulation of muscle contraction	1.53E-02	3	85
angiogenesis	1.65E-02	4	237
regulation of muscle cell apoptotic process	1.69E-02	2	15
negative regulation of epithelial to mesenchymal transition	1.69E-02	2	15
aorta development	1.69E-02	2	15
regulation of ossification	1.81E-02	3	91
regulation of transcription regulatory region DNA binding	1.87E-02	2	16
trabecula morphogenesis	1.87E-02	2	16
muscle cell apoptotic process	1.87E-02	2	16
negative regulation of osteoblast differentiation	2.33E-02	2	18
endocardial cushion development	2.33E-02	2	18
embryonic placenta development	2.33E-02	2	18
regulation of muscle system process	2.48E-02	3	103
cell surface receptor signaling pathway involved in heart develop-ment	2.57E-02	2	19
developmental growth	3.14E-02	3	112
negative regulation of muscle cell differentiation	3.42E-02	2	22
response to hypoxia	3.43E-02	3	116
response to decreased oxygen levels	3.58E-02	3	118
response to oxygen levels	3.74E-02	3	120
negative regulation of cell morphogenesis involved in differentia-tion	3.97E-02	2	24
positive regulation of stem cell proliferation	4.25E-02	2	25
negative regulation of DNA binding	4.25E-02	2	25
epithelial tube morphogenesis	4.50E-02	3	129
tube morphogenesis	5.00E-02	3	134
ventricular cardiac muscle tissue morphogenesis	5.59E-02	2	29
ventricular cardiac muscle tissue development	5.59E-02	2	29
ossification	5.91E-02	3	143
artery morphogenesis	5.91E-02	2	30
chromatin binding	6.35E-02	3	147

embryonic limb morphogenesis	6.61E-02	2	32
embryonic appendage morphogenesis	6.61E-02	2	32
negative regulation of protein binding	6.90E-02	2	33
regulation of stem cell proliferation	6.90E-02	2	33
artery development	6.90E-02	2	33
placenta development	7.67E-02	2	35
regulation of kidney development	7.67E-02	2	35
glomerulus development	9.47E-02	2	39
endothelial cell differentiation	9.90E-02	2	40

FDR: False discovery rate is greater than or equal to the probability that thus is false positive.

Table (5): The genes co-expressed and share a domain with *GATA 4* (7)

Gene 1	Gene 2	Weight	Network group
BMP7	GATA4	0.027017	Co-expression
HEY2	GATA4	0.023368	Co-expression
NKX2-5	GATA4	0.016262	Co-expression
BMP5	GATA4	0.015497	Co-expression
GIP	GATA4	0.0142	Co-expression
JARID2	GATA4	0.014064	Co-expression
GATA6	GATA4	0.010968	Co-expression
GATA5	GATA4	0.010195	Co-expression
CHRD	GATA4	0.007406	Co-expression
SRF	GATA4	0.408248	Genetic interactions
GIP	GATA4	0.475963	Pathway
HEY2	GATA4	0.407109	Pathway
HEY1	GATA4	0.254213	Pathway
BMP10	GATA4	0.080991	Pathway
BMP5	GATA4	0.075797	Pathway
BMP7	GATA4	0.063927	Pathway
SRF	GATA4	0.06354	Pathway
CHRD	GATA4	0.062817	Pathway
NOG	GATA4	0.062817	Pathway
SMAD6	GATA4	0.061585	Pathway
NKX2-5	GATA4	0.060469	Pathway

TBX5	GATA4	1.133502	Physical interactions
JARID2	GATA4	0.801346	Physical interactions
NKX2-5	GATA4	0.741496	Physical interactions
HAMP	GATA4	0.420275	Physical interactions
COL1A2	GATA4	0.406272	Physical interactions
SRF	GATA4	0.245554	Physical interactions
NKX2-5	GATA4	0.909516	Predicted
ZFPM1	GATA4	0.859532	Predicted
SMARCD3	GATA4	0.673114	Predicted
THAP11	GATA4	0.330763	Predicted
JARID2	GATA4	0.107665	Predicted
GATA5	GATA4	0.398371	Shared protein domains
GATA6	GATA4	0.314221	Shared protein domains

DISCUSSION

nsSNPs in coding region:

We compared between wild and mutant residue which is differ on size, charge, domain and hydrophobicity value in six highest deleterious SNPs:

The wild residue of **rs56298569** SNP is neutral, the mutant residue is negatively charged. This can cause repulsion between the mutant residue and neighboring residues, the wild-type residue is much conserved, but a few other residue types have been observed at this position too. Mutant residue is located near a highly conserved position. Based on conservation scores this mutation is probably damaging to the protein. It should be noticed that this residue is also part of an interpro domain named Zinc Finger, Nhr/gata-Type (IPR013088). More broadly speaking, these GO annotations indicate the domain has a function in Ion Binding (GO: 0043167). The mutated residue is located in a domain that is important for binding of other molecules. The mutated residue is in contact with residues in another domain. It is possible that the mutation disturbs these contacts.

The mutant residue of **rs138404762** SNP is bigger than the wild-type residue. The wild-type residue is positively charged, the mutant residue is neutral. The mutant residue is more hydrophobic than the wild-type residue. The residue is located on the surface of the protein; mutation of this residue can disturb interactions with other molecules or other parts of the protein. In addition mutant residue is located near a highly conserved position. But the wild-type residue is not conserved at this position. The other residue type is not similar to mutant residue. Therefore, the mutation is possibly damaging. Also this residue is part of an interpro domain named Transcription Factor Gata-4/gata-Binding Factor A (IPR028436).The mutated residue is located in a domain that is important for binding of other molecules and in contact with residues in a domain that is also important for binding. The mutation might disturb the interaction between these two domains and as such affect the function of the protein.

The mutant residue of **rs180765750** SNP is smaller than the wild-type residue. The wild-type residue is positively charged, the mutant residue is neutral. The wild-type residue is much conserved, but a few other residue types have been observed at this position too. Mutant residue was among the residues at this position observed in other sequences. This means that homologous proteins exist with the same residue type as mutant at this position and this mutation is possibly not damaging to the protein.

The mutant residue of **rs267601735** SNP is smaller than the wild-type residue. The wild-type residue is much conserved, but a few other residue types have been observed at this position too. Based on conservation scores this mutation is probably damaging to the protein. In addition mutant residue is located near a highly conserved position. This will cause a possible loss of external interactions.

The mutant residue of **rs377222076** SNP is bigger than the wild-type residue. The wild-type residue was neutral, the mutant residue is positively charged. The wild-type residue is more hydrophobic than the mutant residue. The wild-type residue occurs often at this position in the sequence, but other residues have also been observed here. On other hand mutant residue is among the other residue types that have been observed at this position in homologous sequences. This means that this mutation can occur at this position and is probably not damaging to the protein.

The mutant residue of **rs387906771** SNP is bigger than the wild-type residue. The mutant residue is more hydrophobic than the wild-type residue. The wild-type residue is much conserved, but a few other residue types have been observed at this position too. Neither your mutant residue nor another residue type with similar properties was observed at this position in other homologous sequences. Based on conservation scores this mutation is probably damaging to the protein and mutant residue is located near a highly conserved position.

SNPs in 3' UTR region:

We found 164 functional classes in 34 SNPs at 3' UTR region; 55 were 'D' allele D' allele that disrupts a conserved miRNA site and 99 were 'C' allele as target binging site can be disrupts a conserved miRNA. **RS1062221** contained 14 'C' allele as target binging site can be disrupts a conserved miRNA and one 'D' allele while **rs146304341** had 12 'D' allele that disrupts a conserved miRNA site and 7 'C' allele.

SNP in 5' UTR region:

We found one SNP namely **rs61277615** was located at a transcription factor-binding site (TFBS) of a gene may affect the level, location, or timing of gene expression and also not have exonic splicing enhancer (ESE), or exonic splicing silencer (ESS) to disrupt splicing activity and cause alternative splicing.

CONCLUSION

In conclusion, our results suggest that the application of computational tools like SIFT, Poly-Phen-2, I mutant-3. Phd-SNP, polymRTS, SNP Function Prediction and Project Hope may provide an alternative approach for selecting target SNPs. The *GATA-4* gene responsible for causing congenital heart defect especially in newborns was investigated through computational methods and the influence of functional SNPs were evaluated. In a total of 18598 SNPs, 192 were found to be nonsynonymous. Out of the 192 nsSNPs, 29 nsSNPs were found to be deleterious and damaging by SIFT and 22 nsSNPs by PolyPhen server. Twenty two nsSNPs were found to be common in both SIFT and PolyPhen server. Also, 6 nsSNPs were observed to be highly deleterious and damaging as per SIFT and PolyPhen server. Moreover the PolymiRTS results showed 34 SNPs in the 3'UTR region and only one SNP in 5' UTR by SNP Function Prediction to be functionally significant. Hence, we hope our results will provide useful information that needed to help researchers to do further study in heart disease in children especially in our country.

ACKNOWLEDGMENTS

Authors express their deep gratitude to African City of Technology members for their assistance and help.

Competing interests

The authors declare that they have no competing interests.

References

1. Garg V. Insights into the genetic basis of congenital heart disease. *Cellular and Molecular Life Sciences CMLS.* 2006; 63(10):1141-8.

2. Ransom J, Srivastava D. The genetics of cardiac birth defects. *Semin Cell Dev Biol.* 2007;18(1):132-9.

3. Marelli AJ, Mackie AS, Ionescu-Ittu R, Rahme E, Pilote L. Congenital heart disease in the general populationchanging prevalence and age distribution. *Circulation.* 2007; 115(2):163-72.

4. Misra C, Sachan N, McNally CR, Koenig SN, Nichols HA, Guggilam A. *et.al.* Congenital heart disease-causing Gata4 mutation displays functional deficits in vivo. *PLoS Genet.* 2012; 8(5):e1002690.

5. Frey N, Katus HA. Dilated cardiomyopathy as a genetic disease: molecular and clinical aspects. *Internist (Berl).*2008, 49:43-50.

6. Humbert M, Nunes H, Sitbon O. *et. al.* Risk factors for pulmonary arterial hypertension. *Clin Chest Med.* 2001; 22(3):459 -75.

7. Schork NJ, Fallin D, Lanchbury S. Single nucleotide polymorphisms and the future of genetic epidemiology. *Clin Genet.* 2000; 58(4): 250–64.

8. Kwok PY, Chen X. Detection of Single Nucleotide Polymorphisms. *Curr. Issues Mol. Biol.*2003; 5: 43-60.

9. Bao L, Cui Y. Functional impacts of non-synonymous single nucleotide polymorphisms: Selective constraint and structural environments. *FEBS Letters* 2006; 580(5): 1231–34.

10 Arceci RJ, King A, Simon MC, Orkin SH, Wilson DB. Mouse GATA-4: a retinoic acid-inducible GATA-binding transcription factor expressed in endodermally derived tissues and heart. *Molec. Cell. Biol.*1993; 13(4): 2235-46.

11. Sunagawa Y, Katanasaka Y, Wada H, Hasegawa K, Morimoto T. Functional Analysis of GATA4 Complex, a Cardiac Hypertrophy-response Transcriptional Factor, Using a Proteomics Approach. *Yakugaku Zasshi.* 2015; 136(2):151-6.

12. Liu XY, Wang J, Zheng JH, Bai K, Liu ZM, Wang XZ, *et al*. Involvement of a novel GATA4 mutation in atrial septal defects. *Int J Mol Med*. 2011; 28(1):17–23.

13. Pu WT, Ishiwata T, Juraszek AL, Ma Q and Izumo S. GATA4 is a dosage-sensitive regulator of cardiac morphogenesis. *Dev Biol*. 2004; 275(1): 235-244.

14. Zeisberg EM, Ma Q, Juraszek AL, Moses K, Schwartz RJ, Izumo S, Pu WT. Morphogenesis of the right ventricle requires myocardial expression of Gata4. *J Clin Invest*. 2005; 115(6):1522-31.

15. Xin M, Davis CA, Molkentin JD, Lien CL, Duncan SA, Richardson JA and Olson EN (2006). A threshold of GATA4 and GATA6 expression is required for cardiovascular development. *Proc Natl Acad Sci*. 2006; 103(30): 11189-94.

16. Rivera-Feliciano J, Lee KH, Kong SW, Rajagopal S, Ma Q, Springer Z, Izumo S, Tabin CJ, Pu WT. Development of heart valves requires Gata4 expression in endothelial-derived cells. *Development*. 2006; 133(18):3607-18.

17. Maitra M, Schluterman MK, Nichols HA, Richardson JA, Lo CW, Srivastava D, Garg V. Interaction of Gata4 and Gata6 with Tbx5 is critical for normal cardiac development. *Dev Biol*. 2009; 326(2):368-77.

18. Bentham J, Bhattacharya S.Genetic mechanisms controlling cardiovascular development. *Ann N Y Acad Sci*. 2008; 1123(1):10-9.

19. Watt AJ, Battle MA, Li J, Duncan SA.GATA4 is essential for formation of the proepicardium and regulates cardiogenesis. *Proc Natl Acad Sci*. 2004; 101(34):12573-8.

20. Huang WY, Cukerman E, Liew CC. Identification of a GATA motif in the cardiac α-myosin heavy-chain-encoding gene and isolation of a human GATA-4 cDNA. *Gene*. 1995; 155(2):219-23.

21. Garg V, Kathiriya IS, Barnes R, Schluterman MK, King IN, Butler CA, Rothrock CR, Eapen RS, Hirayama-Yamada K, Joo K, Matsuoka R. GATA4 mutations cause human congenital heart defects and reveal an interaction with TBX5. *Nature*. 2003; 424(6947):443-7.

22. Rojas A, Kong SW, Agarwal P, Gilliss B, Pu WT, Black BL. GATA4 is a direct transcriptional activator of cyclin D2 and Cdk4 and is required for cardiomyocyte proliferation in anterior heart field-derived myocardium. *J Mol Cell Biol*. 2008;28(17):5420-31.

23. Rajagopal SK, Ma Q, Obler D, Shen J, Manichaikul A, Tomita-Mitchell A. *et. al.* Spectrum of heart disease associated with murine and human GATA4 mutation. J Mol Cell Cardiol. 2007; 43(6):677-85.

24. Sarkozy A, Conti E, Neri C, d'Agostino R, Digilio MC, Esposito G, *et. al.* Spectrum of atrial septal defects associated with mutations of NKX2. 5 and GATA4 transcription factors J Med Genet. 2005; 42(2):e16-.

25. Ng PC, Henikoff S. SIFT: Predicting amino acid changes that affect protein function. *Nucleic Acids Res.*. 2003;31(13):3812-4.

26. Ramensky V, Bork P, Sunyaev S. Human non-synonymous SNPs: server and survey. *Nucleic Acids Res*. 2002;30(17):3894-900.

27. Capriotti E, Fariselli P, Rossi I, Casadio R. A three-state prediction of single point mutations on protein stability changes. *BMC bioinformatics*. 2008;9(2):1. DOI: 10.1186/1471-2105-9-S12-S6

28. Capriotti E, Calabrese R, Casadio R. Predicting the insurgence of human genetic diseases associated to single point protein mutations with support vector machines and evolutionary information. *Bioinformatics*. 2006;22(22):2729-34.

29. Venselaar H, te Beek TA, Kuipers RK, Hekkelman ML, Vriend G. Protein structure analysis of mutations causing inheritable diseases. An e-Science approach with life scientist friendly interfaces. BMC bioinformatics. 2010;11(1):1. DOI: 10.1186/1471-2105-11-548. PubMed: 21059217.

30 Jia M, Yang B, Li Z, Shen H, Song X, Gu W. Computational analysis of functional single nucleotide polymorphisms associated with the CYP11B2 gene. *PloS one*. 2014;9(8):e104311. DOI:10.1371/journal.pone.0104311

31. Osman MM, Khalifa AS, Mutasim AEY, Massaad SO, Gasemelseed MM, Abdagader MA, *et al.* In Silico Analysis of Single Nucleotide Polymorphisms (Snps) in Human FTO Gene. *J Bioinform, Genomics, Proteomics.2016;* 1(1): 1003.

32. Warde-Farley D, Donaldson SL, Comes O, Zuberi K, Badrawi R, Chao P, *et. al.* The GeneMANIA prediction server: biological network integration for gene prioritization and predicting gene function. Nucleic Acids Res. 2010; 38(suppl 2):W214-20.

YOUR KNOWLEDGE HAS VALUE

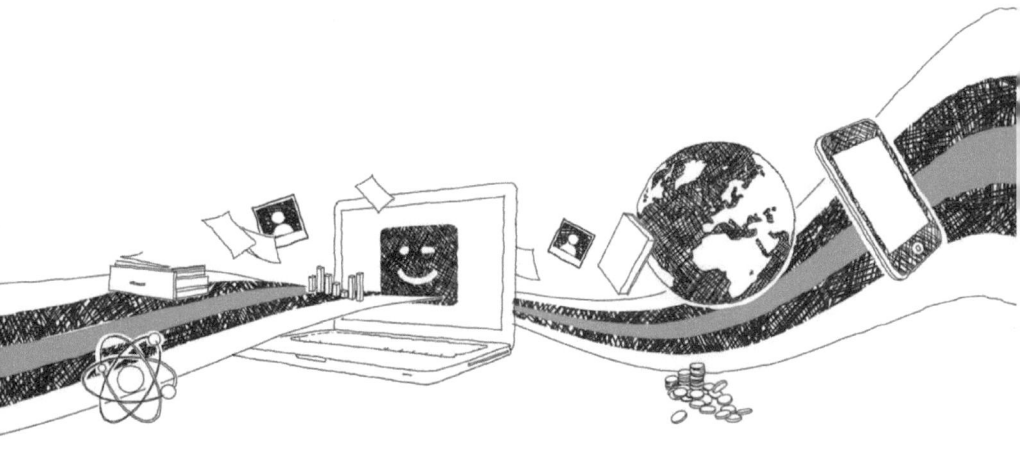

- We will publish your bachelor's and
  master's thesis, essays and papers

- Your own eBook and book -
  sold worldwide in all relevant shops

- Earn money with each sale

Upload your text at www.GRIN.com
and publish for free

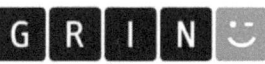